Dedicated to ALL MY CLIENTS past and present

Disclaimer

With Anita's skin care knowledge, by no means makes her a specialist. This guide is to share her knowledge to the reader and not to dictate, assume information is suitable or aimed at all situations.
This guide is for educational and entertainment purposes only. Every attempt has been made to provide accurate, up to date and reliable information. No warranties of any kind are expressed or implied.
Readers acknowledge that the author is not engaging in the rendering of legal, financial, medical or professional advice.
This Guide is to help the reader in their day to day skin care routines and helps identify various skin care issues and ailments.

By reading this Guide, the reader agrees that under no circumstances is Anita responsible for any losses, direct or indirect which are incurred as a result of the use of information contained within this guide, including, but not limited to, errors, omissions, or inaccuracies.

ISBN #: 978-1-716-960-475

Author Biography:

Anita E. Viljoen graduated M Beautician School in 2008 and received her Cosmetology Institute (BC Council) Certification in 2009. She has been a licensed member of the BC Beauty Council ever since. Being an Aesthetician and working on various clients young and old skin for over 10 years has given her extensive knowledge to skin care.

Beauty Council History (taken from https://www.beautycouncil.ca/cpages/about)

For almost 90 years BeautyCouncil, the former Hairdressing Association of BC and Cosmetology Association of BC, was a provincial government regulated body for the cosmetology industry. When government regulation ceased in 2003, the industry created a voluntary association comprised of caring, driven and committed professionals who recognized a need for industry standards to be upheld.
Today we continue to oversee the growth and development of training, certification, advocacy and events for Western Canada's beauty professionals. We are a member driven non-profit organization that fosters private sector partnerships, advances the interests of the industry and raises professional standards.

My Reflection

I often find myself looking at my reflection in the mirror, like most of us do, and wonder why my skin looks the way it does? When did I age? When did the years start showing up around my eyes? Using my fingers to lift the soft skin around my sunken eyes, dark and swollen, they did not look like this a few years ago. I am sure, felt like yesterday, they were bright and firm.

I was blessed with healthy skin, with the occasional teenage breakout. My mother believed in *Oil of Olay®* so that was my first skin care routine; Cleanser, Toner and Moisturizer with *clearasil®* for the breakouts.
Not everyone may have the genes, routines and knowledge to help them through their acne and aging skin issues. I have the genes, the routines and much later on in life I administered the knowledge.

As an esthetician my knowledge to skin disorders are limited and can only recommend professional and clinical products available to me. I have shared what works with many of my clients and when I come across something perplex, I take the time to research and find the best way to treat them. Some cases, not many, doctors need to step in to help. I don't always agree with the chemical, pharmaceutical approach, I tend to lean more toward naturopathic and alternative ways in solving acne, ageing and skin issues.
I also have a strong belief in what you put into your mouth will affect your bodies reaction to it.
Food is best from a plant, not made in a plant. Grass and free range fed animal meat are healthiest.

This is why I have created this guide to assist.

Chapter One - Your Skin

Before we get started with your skin care routines and what products to use and why, we need to understand how your skin works.
This brings awareness of any changes and problems that may arise and how to treat it.

As you know skin is the largest organ of the body, which is made of cells, which holds 60% to 90% of water.

Healthy skin is plump, soft, smooth and with a perfect Ph balance.

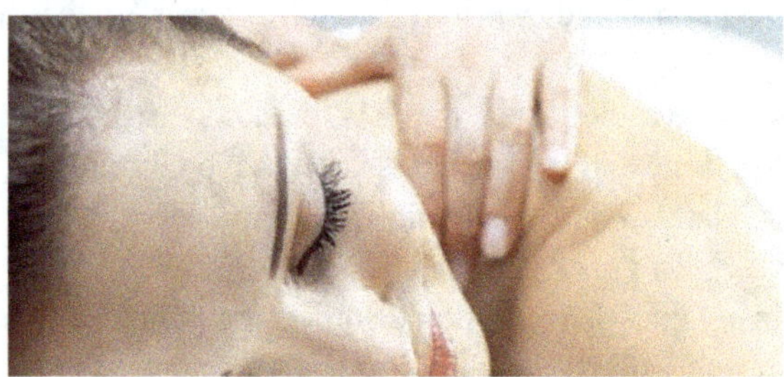

Skin pH Balance

Your skin pH balance is important, any changes to this balance may cause reactions.

The **pH level** of the **skin** refers to how acidic or alkaline it is. On a scale of 1-14, with 1 being the most acidic to 14 being the most alkaline. Our **skin** has a thin, protective layer on its surface, referred to as the acid mantle.

When it comes to the **pH** of your **skin**, it's reliant on the skin's acid mantle. This acid mantle protects **skin** against external influences like bad bacteria, allergens and pollution, while maintaining moisture. For your **skin** to remain **balanced**, your acid mantle will naturally stay slightly acidic with a **pH** of around 4.5 to 5.5.

The following Factors can affect skin pH balance include:
- Air pollution
- Antibacterial soaps and gels
- Change in seasons (different humidity)
- Cosmetics
- Detergents
- Sebum/ skin moisture
- Sweat
- TAP WATER (including too frequent washing / exfoliation of skin)
- Too much sun exposure

Microbiome

The **microbiome** is a community of living micro-organisms made up of mostly bacteria, but can also contain fungi, viruses, and mites. It works to protect the **skin** and keep the **skin** barrier functioning.

Skin Biology

Skin layers, nerves, cellular functions, hair follicles and glands.

Skin Layers: **Epidermis** the outermost layer of skin composed of _5 cellular layers_ all surrounded by Lipids which is best explained as an intercellular cement which helps cells from water loss and provides hydration.

1. Outermost layer which is our primary concern. Also known as the horny layer because of the scale-like cells made primarily of soft

Keratin. **Keratin** is a fiber protein that provides resiliency and protection to the skin (Hard Keratin is found in hair and nails).
Keratin is continually shedding and replacing – this is called cell turnover which we will talk more about in this chapter.

2. The next layer is a clear layer made of small cells that lets light pass through, this layer is only found on the palms of the hands and soles of the feet, acts like a barrier.

3. The third layer resembles granules, which are filled with Keratin and also produces lipids. These move to the surface to shed off.

4. The fourth layer is a spiny layer this assist in holding cells together.

5. Fifth layer is also known as the basal layer and the first layer just above the Dermis.

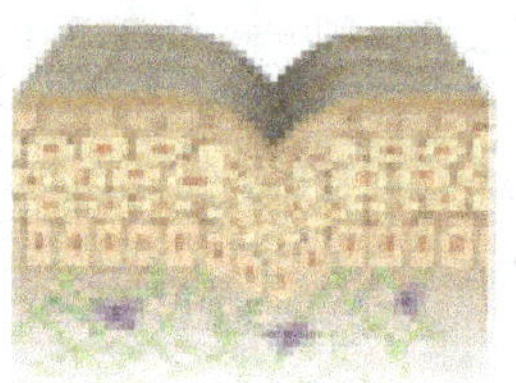 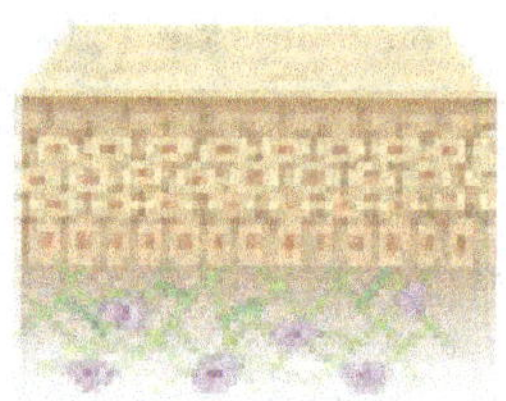

The Dermis composes of _2 live layers_ of connective tissues 25 times thicker than the epidermis layers. These layers hold blood, lymph vessels which supplies nourishment, oil, sweat glands, nerves and arrector pili (this is responsible for goosebumps).

1. Papillary Layer is found as small cone-shaped structures which contains hair follicles that is nourished by blood and nerve endings.

2. Reticular layer is the deepest layer of the Dermis contains protein fibers, that gives the skin strength and elasticity, **Collagen** are produced by fibroblast and makes up 70% of the Dermis. In contrast 2.5% of **Elastin** is found in the dermis.
Damage or break down to these fibers are the primary cause of wrinkles and aging.
Also, between these fibers, **hyaluronic acid** is found.

** Ingredients replicated to match these natural fluids are the focus of products development today in the anti-aging industry – will be discussed in page 32.

2.a. At the bottom of the Reticular layer is composed of fat tissue this protective cushion gives contour and smoothness to the body and a great source of energy. This layer decreases with age.

Cell Replacement:

The body replaces billions of cells daily, organs such as the skin, heart, liver and kidneys constantly have their cells replaced every six to nine months.
Unfortunately, **elastin and collagen** are not replaced naturally by the body alone and the skin does not regain its once-firm shape after being stretched and expanded over time. However, research shows certain products and ingredients stimulate collagen and elastin growth.

Cell regeneration slows down with the production of Collagen and Elastin.
Ages 9 to 19 your cells regenerate up to 7 days;
Ages 20 to 25 your cells regenerate within 10 to 14 days;

Ages 26 to 35 your cells regenerate within 14 – 21 days, at this time Collagen production slows down;
Ages 36 to 45 your cells regenerate within 15 – 25 days, Collagen and Elastin production slows down even more.
Ages 46 to 65 your cells regenerate within 25 – 30 days, no Collagen and Elastin production;
Ages 66 to 90 your cells regenerate very slowly, depends on health - medications, hormones and environmental influences will influence your skin and organ repair.

Skin Colour:

Cells that produce pigment granules in the basal layers is called melanocytes. These granules produce a complex protein, melanin which determine skin and hair colour. **Melanin** is transferred into the cells that move up to the skins surface. It also protects the cells below from ultraviolet rays by absorbing and blocking UV rays through tanning.

Glands:

Two types of duct glands located in the dermis of the skin;

1. Oil (sebaceous) glands secretes oil which is connected to the hair follicles, these ducts can become clogged and pimples are formed. Oil glands are larger on the face and scalp.
These clogged glands can also cause hair to become ingrown.

2 Sweat (sudoriferous) glands secretes sweat to regulate body temperature.

With skin replacement (regeneration) it is important to know when you injure yourself or find you have compromised the skin's PH balance, how fast the skin will repair with the knowledge above.
You may need to help your skin do this by addressing the problem yourself or some cases, your esthetician or in server cases, your doctor.

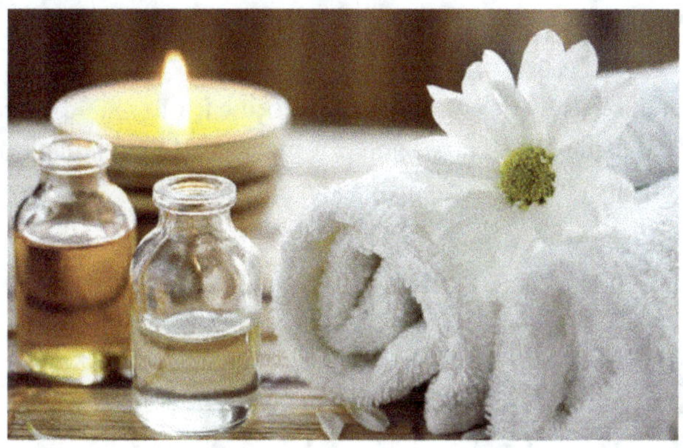

Chapter Two – Skin Routines

The practice of self-grooming and beautification has been found in ancient cultures often allied with the practice of medicine.
Egyptians have used personal grooming regiments by using herbal and flower essences, which is still the preferred method of extracting essential oils today. The Egyptians believed in cleanliness and built elaborate systems for bathing which were later adopted by the Greek and Romans.

Asian and African ancient grooming traced back to 2900 B.C.E. both originated using herbal cures and raw materials found in their natural environments (soil, insects, plants and animals).

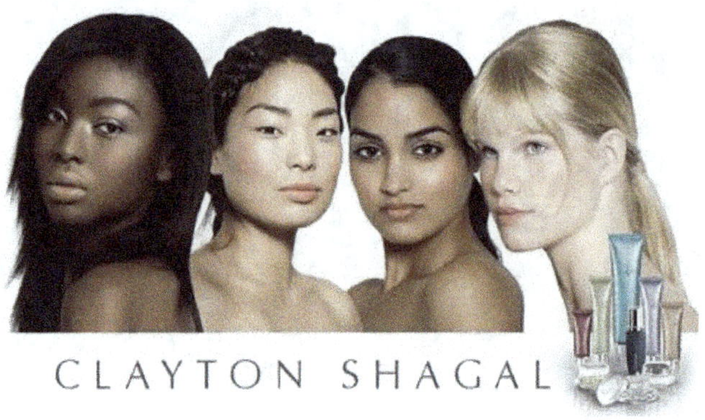

Your Routine

Daily bathing/showering is important way in protecting ourselves from infections, illnesses and ailments and maintain good health. It also important for our self-confidence, physical and emotional well-being. The main purpose is to removal dirt and odours, left behind by sweat and oils (sebum).

Washing your skin with warm to <u>hot water</u> is important as it releases dirt and oils imbedded in the pores. It also allows blood to rise up to the skin surface, which helps supply the skin with nutrients, oxygen and removes waste. Rinse with tepid to <u>cold water</u> is advised to slow down the blood supply (redness to the skin).

It is important to know, pores are not like elastic bands that open and close at will. Pores increase in size due to oil and dirt building up in them, which expands the look of them. It takes time and a good routine to reduce and keep pores healthy.

Steps to healthy skin

I would recommend following the steps your esthetician prescribes for you and your skin type, however there are three general steps.

- Step one – cleanse and rinse with warm water.
- Step two – cleanse again (some cases use a gentle exfoliator) and rinse with cold water / then use a toner.
- Step three – moisturize.

These general steps may be necessary twice a day, morning and night.

Young to pre-teen youth routine -
<u>Evenings only:</u>

Pea size amount and rub in **Cleanser** - rinse
Use pea size amount of **Moisturize**, apply to face.

Teen to young Adult with combination skin:
<u>Morning and Evenings</u>

1. Pea size amount and rub in **Cleanser** - rinse.

2. Add **Scrub** twice a week to your routine to remove dead skin cells and debris.

3. Use pea size amount of **Moisturizer**, apply to face.

Acne prone skin
Morning and Evenings

1. Peas size amount of **Purifying Cleanser** - Rinse,
2. **Scrub** - Rinse.
3. On dry clean skin pat on **Elastin Gel** (use spatula, not finger)
4. Use pea size amount of **Moisturizer**, apply to face.

Adult - Due to loss of Collagen and Hydration in our skin as from 25 years onward, this is your routine in variations

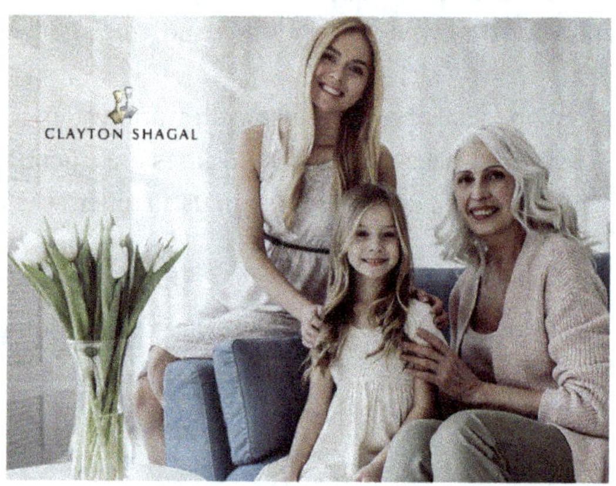

Mornings

1. Peas size amount of **Cleanser,** rinse
2. On dry clean skin, pat on **Collagen Gel** (use spatula, not finger to remove from jar) dry, clean skin
3. One pump of **Hyaluronic Acid** and apply to area's needing more moisture.
4. Finish off with a **Moisturizer**

Evenings
1. Peas size amount of **Cleanser,** rinse.
2. Twice a week add **Scrub** to your routine to keep remove dead skin cells and debris.
3. On dry clean skin, pat on **Elastin Gel** (use spatula, not finger to remove from jar) dry, clean skin
4. One pump of **Hyaluronic Acid** and apply to area's needing more moisture (under eye's).
5. Finish off with **Moisturizer**.
** Tip: add a pump of Hyaluronic Acid to the Moisturizer

Never go to bed with make-up on!!

Make-Up:

Sleeping in your make-up every now and again will not do too much harm, however routinely:

1. Doing so will age your skin faster due to breakdown of the make-up itself can prevent the important role of microcirculation, which helps renew the skin. These speeds the breakdown of collagen, resulting in wrinkles. Waking up with aged, stressed and dull skin.

2. It blocks pores, leaving oil trapped inside, this leads to bacteria build up, breakouts and enlarged pores, yes all of them.

3. Lose your eyelashes – left on mascara can cause eyelashes to become brittle and weak and can break easily and even shed faster.

4. Eye infections and cysts can become a double disaster.

Please take the time to wash your face before you go to bed, make it a part of your routine, your skin will be healthier, younger and clear.

Extra tip - wash your pillow case weekly.

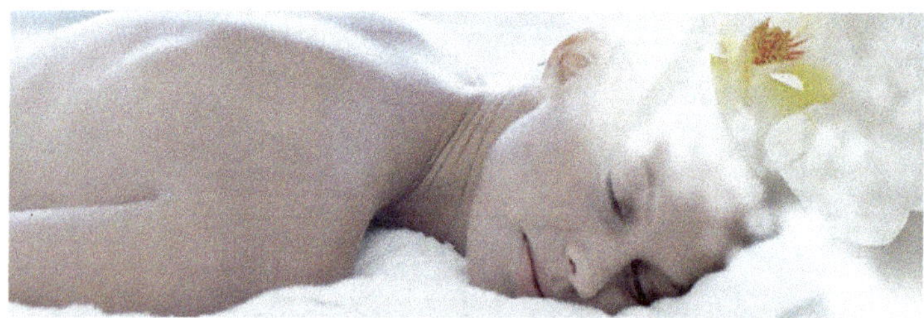

Chapter Three - Acne Prone Skin

Acne can start as young as 9 years old, so the sooner you start with a good skin routine, the better. It is most common at the first sign of puberty, in girls 14 to 17 and boys 15 – 19 years of age and normally disappears by age 25, although 12% of women and 3% of men, have acne until the age of 44 years of age.

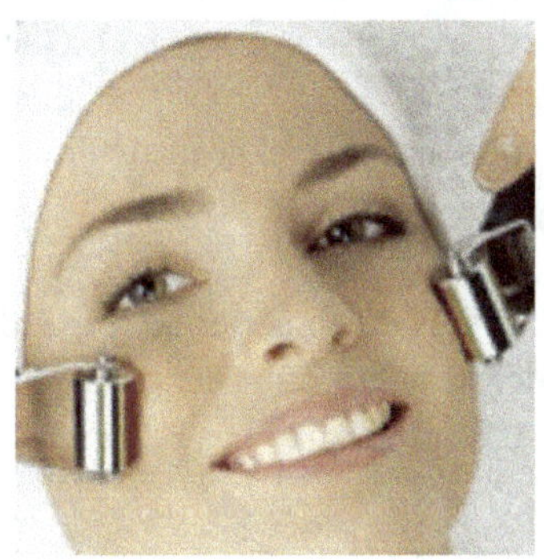

Causes of Acne

Acne, also known as acne vulgaris is a long-term skin disease that occurs when hair follicles are clogged with dead skin cells and oil (sebum).

Genetics is thought to be the primary cause of acne 80% of the time.

The role of diet and smoking can also be the cause of acne, but not medically substantiated, however, I personally found in changing your diet does influence skin allergies causing Acne. We will discuss Diet on Page 28.

Hormones appear to be part of the underlying mechanism, by casing increased production of sebum.

Birth Control may help against acne, while others may cause it. Discuss this with your doctor.

There are various stages, and kinds of Acne, this chapter will explain what the differences are and to understand these stages in severity will help you treat them.

Stage I– Minor breakouts, restricted to whiteheads, blackheads, with a few papules and pustules.

Stage II – moderate acne consists of multiple whiteheads, blackheads, papules and pustules spread to various areas on the body.

Stage III – many whiteheads, blackheads with papules and pustules red and inflamed.

Stage IV – Cystic acne, is the most serious type of acne. It develops when cysts form deep underneath your skin. They are aggressive, painful and found on face, chest and back.

Kinds of Acne

Most Acne is <u>not</u> caused by dirt. Usually made out of Keratin (skin debris, hair and sebum).

Whiteheads are clogged oil trapped in duct the pore, closed.

Blackheads are made of clogged oil trapped in the top of the pore, open, that has oxidized.

Papules a pimple; small elevation on the skin that contains no fluid, but may develop pus.

Pustules are inflamed pus (bacterial or fungal) topically found with a white or yellow head.

Sebaceous filaments are a tiny collection of sebum and dead skin cells around a hair follicle, which usually takes the form of a small hair-like strand. They usually have white or yellow colour and can be expressed from the skin by pinching. These filaments are naturally occurring and are not a sign of infection.

Cystic Acne are aggressive, inflamed, painful or tender to the touch, they are pus-filled cysts, large white to red bumps deep in the skin. Does not come to a head and often red and swollen.

Milia are tiny, pearl-like bumps, hard to the touch, they are not acne.

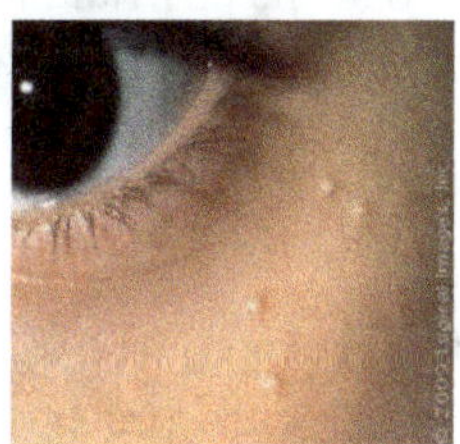

Unlike acne, milia are rather firm, and squeezing has little to no impact on them, these bumps may show up around the eyes and on parts of the face where there aren't active oil glands. Milia also don't have the pain associated with it, unlike acne when a pimple forms and then becomes inflamed and sore.

Milia occur when dead skin cells get trapped under the skin's surface, forming small, hard cysts.

Adults can get two forms of milia: primary and secondary.
- Primary is the type also seen in babies, caused by skin cells that build up and does not exfoliate properly.

- Secondary milia happens when a skin condition that leads to blistering actually damages the pore lining. Burns or severe rashes can increase the number of skin cells trapped under the skin's surface.

Sun damage is also a contributing factor to milia because it makes skin rough and leathery, so it's more difficult for dead cells to rise to the skin's surface and shed normally.

Primarily, it is critical that you not squeeze, scrape, poke, or in any other way physically try to remove the milia from your face as you would a pimple. Instead, you wind up irritating and damaging the skin surrounding the cyst. Some people have even scarred themselves trying to dig out milia—and there's no question a scar will last longer than any milia bump!

Of course, you can see a skin expert, who can tell you which type of milia you have. Secondary milia might require the use of a hypodermic needle to remove the cyst, or cryotherapy. If your milia don't respond to an exfoliating treatment after several weeks, consider making an appointment with your aesthetician or dermatologist.

Cholesterol Build up: If you have yellowish bumps around your eyes and on your eyelids, they are typically translucent flesh to white. You may be dealing with a skin growth known as a xanthoma. These bumps are common in people who have high cholesterol or high triglyceride levels.

Chapter Four - Acne Home Treatment:

ACNE:

- To prevent oil buildup the face should be washed morning and evening with warm to hot water with a mild, gentle nonabrasive cleanser.
- Washing is recommended with the use of your fingers, the use of a washcloth, mesh sponge or anything else that can irritate the skin should be avoided.
- Using a gentle, alcohol- free, Acid-free cleanser, is best. The use of astringents, toners and exfoliants can irritate and dry the skin, making the acne look worse.
- Scrubbing is not helpful; it does not stop acne and can aggravate it.

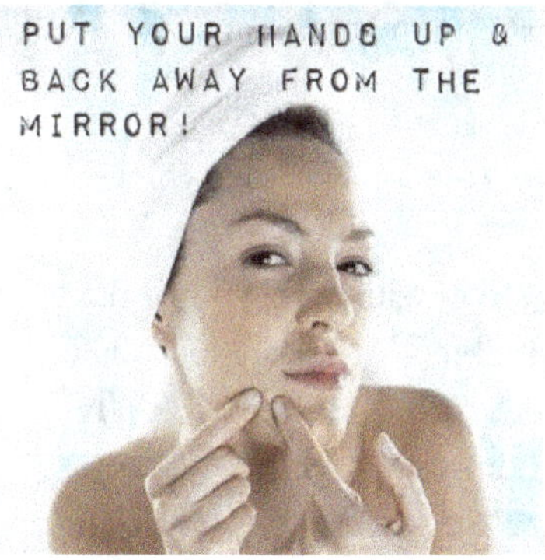

MILIA:

- Although not a lot can be done to prevent milia, they are known to go away on their own without treatment, be patient, however waiting is not for everyone.
- To maintain a suitable skin-care routine certainly helps minimize the chance of them appearing.

- Because secondary milia can be caused by sun damage, always use a moisturizer with at least SPR 15 to protect your skin every day, and give those annoying white bumps less of a reason to set up shop on your face!

Yes, milia is a real pain to put up with, but there are things you can do to treat it. Remember; patience, daily exfoliation, sun protection, and resisting the temptation to take matters into your own hands can go a long way to having clearer, bump-free skin sooner!

Acne Medications and Creams:

Over the Counter / on line treatments for acne are not as effective as one would think. Most cases they start off that way, due to your attention to the skin.
Most of these products contain, alcohols, acids or peroxides that dry out the skin so severely that the bacteria, causing most acne, die. Unfortunately, this is short lived.

Using these products:

- Day One: Skin will feel tight and flakey.
- Day Two: Skin starts drying out and clear up.
- Day Three: Skin clears up and find it gets oily to the touch by late afternoon.
- Day Four: The skin is now overproducing oil, trying to get the pH balance back to normal.
- Day Five: Your skin starts going red, inflamed and in some cases, acne comes back aggressively deep in the skin.

Using the alcohol, acid or peroxide based product will now burn your skin, you may find your skin welt, go raw or become very oily.

What a spiteful cycle.

AS DISCUSSED BEFORE – Keep your Skin pH level between 5.5 - 5.7

**I always recommend a good skin care routine and keep Witch Hazel® with you to tone down the skin after exercise or excessive sweating.

Isotretinoin

Also known as Accutane®, a powerful prescription medication is considered the most effective treatment measure for cystic acne.
It is derived from a powerful vitamin A, taken in tablet form.
About 85 percent of people who take it will experience improvements within four to six months.

There are some serious risks associated with isotretinoin:
- New or worsening mood disorders;
- Inflammatory bowel disease;
- Persistent headaches or nosebleeds;
- Bruising or skin inflammation;
- Blood in your urine;
- Muscle and joint pain;
- kidney issues.

Oral antibiotics

These work by decreasing bacteria and inflammation that could be contributing to cystic acne, but does not alleviate excess oil and dead skin cell production.

Antibiotics should only be used short term, due to over bacterial resistance.

Possible side effects of oral antibiotics may include:
- Abdominal pain
- Diarrhea
- Nausea, to vomiting
- Sun sensitivity

Topical Retinoids

Also derived from vitamin A, these don't have quite the strength of isotretinoin. These work by unplugging hair follicles to remove and prevent severe acne.

Retinoids are used in conjunction with topical antibiotics to make them more effective, on a daily basis as a cream, gels or lotions.

Using topical retinoids can make your skin red and can also cause it to peel. These side effects are usually temporary as your skin gets used to the medication.

Retinoids can also make you more susceptible to sunburn and thins skin down so much that can cause trauma.

** I advised not to use Wax (hair removal) on your skin, while using Retinoid creams.

Spironolactone

Is another possible prescription treatment for cystic acne. Traditionally, its used as a diuretic to help tread edema and high blood pressure, in terms of acne, this medication can work by managing excess androgen levels.

Side effects may cause birth defects, so you should not use if planning a pregnancy or have kidney disease.

- Breast tenderness
- Dizziness
- Fatigue
- Headaches
- High blood potassium
- Menstrual irregularities

Oral contraceptives

These are a viable option for cystic acne in some women. This method is effective due to hormone fluctuations related to your menstrual cycle.
Birth control pills contain estrogen which regulate overall hormone levels and possibly reduce acne.
These still may not be appropriate for everyone and if you smoke, have blood clots or trying to get pregnant.

Acne Scarring

To reduce the risk of scarring by leaving all cysts alone, this means you can't ever pick or pop cysts. Picking at them with your nails, will spread the infections.

There are ways you can try to reduce the appearance of Acne scars. However, it is important you treat the active acne first and then address the scars.

Treatments for Acne scares
These include by a professional:
- Chemical peels
- Microdermabrasion
- Laser resurfacing.

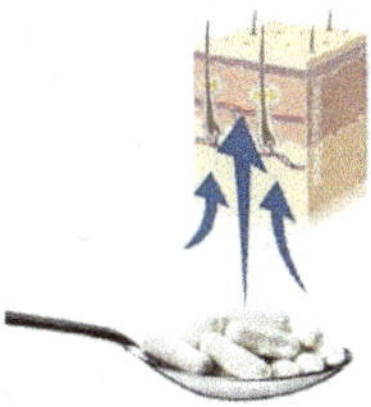

Chapter Five - Other Skin Complications

Rosacea

- A chronic congestion primarily on the cheeks and nose.
- Characterized by redness, dilation of blood vessels, and in server cases papules and pustules can be seen.
- Cause is unknown, but may be due to dryness of the skin and restricted capillaries.
- Aggravation of the condition can be caused by spicy foods, alcohol, caffeine, exposure to extreme temperatures, stress and sun.
- Soothing and calming ingredients and treatments will help calm the skin and decrease the inflammation.

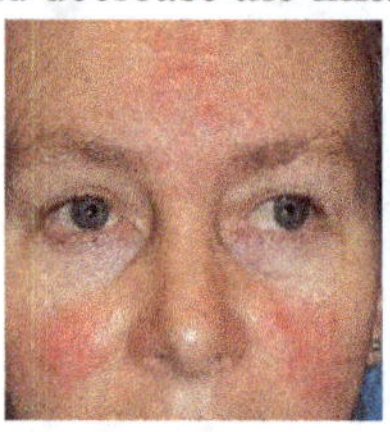

Eczema

Inflammation of the skin with a painful itching, acute or chronic in nature with dry or moist lesions.

Psoriasis

- A skin disease characterized by red patches covered with white silver scales.
- Caused by an over proliferation of skin cells and replicate too fast.
- It is not contagious but can be spread by irritating it.

Skin Cancer

Caused by cumulative sun exposure comes in three distinctive forms varying in severity:

<u>Basal Cell Carcinoma</u> is the most common and the least severe type
of carcinoma.
It appears as light pearly nodules.

<u>Squamous Cell Carcinoma</u> is a more serious condition then Basal.
It appears as scaly red papules or nodules.

<u>Malignant Melanoma</u> is a the most serious form of skin cancer.
Black or dark patches on the skin are usually uneven in texture jagged
or raised.
It is not always found on areas exposed to sunlight.

Chapter Six - Contraindications on Services

What you need to disclose to your esthetician:

Disclosed Contraindications	Affects What services	Reason
Asthma / Sinus / Nasal allergies	Facials	Steam may result breathing problems
Hepatitis	All	Contagious contact pathogens
Metal bone, pins or plates	Facials and Laser	*Electricity, tools may cause Cardiac problems /discomfort
Pacemaker	Laser	In extreme cases can cause heart failure
High Blood Pressure	Facials, Pedicures	May cause dizziness
Epilepsy/ Psychological	Laser	unconsciousness, seizures. Chronic Headaches
Eczema / Psoriasis	All services	Skin irritation, burn, blistering

Herpes / Fever Blisters	All	Contagious
Lupus / Immune disorders	Facials, Waxing	Skin irritation, to severe reactions
Pregnancy	Some Facials, Laser	*Electricity may be threatening to Fetus.

Skin Cancer	Facials, Laser, Waxing	may cause Irritation, aggravation

Medications:	Affects What services	Disclosed Contraindications
Birth control/ Hormone	Facials, Laser, Waxing	May not be as affective
Azelex / Differin / Renova / **Retin-A** Tazarac Glycolic / Alphahydroxy Acids Accutane	Facials, Waxing, Laser	Skin thinning properties may cause skin to tear, blister or bleed.

Chapter Seven - Skin Aging

Approximately 85% of our aging is caused by the rays of the sun. As we age, the collagen and elastin fibers of the skin naturally weaken this happens faster when the skin is exposed   to ultraviolet rays too often.

UVA rays also called the "Aging rays"   contribute 95% of the skins ultraviolet rays that reach the earth's surface these rays weaken the skins collagen and elastin fibers causing wrinkling and sagging.
UVB rays also referred to as the "Burning rays" causes tanning of the skin. Melanin is designed to help protect the skin from the sun UV rays.

On a positive note, UVB rays contribute to the body synthesis of vitamin D, important minerals and energy. Early morning sun exposure is highly recommended.

Environment: While sun may play a predominate role in how the skin ages, pollutants in the air from factories, cars and overall health of our skin can affect the surface of the skin health.

According to dermatologist; Your skin breaks down during the day due to exposure to the environmental pollutants as well as bacteria, molds, mites from the outside.

Signs of Aging

There are key signs of Aging:
- Fine lines and Wrinkles,
- Dullness,
- Uneven skin tone, Blotchiness and Age Spots
- Dryness, Rough texture,
- Sagging skin, loss of volume and elasticity.

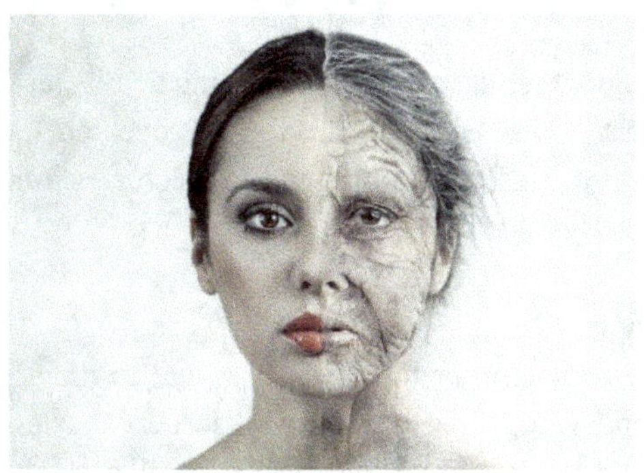

Key signs of Premature Aging:

- Your outlook and perception;
  The mind plays a significant role in whether we are aging faster or slower, and we can use the mind help us accelerate or decelerate the process. Research found happier people are quite simply younger looking people.

- Smoking and Drinking;
  We know doing so in excess are not good for us in general, this leads to all kinds of health problems as necessary nutrients are restricted to hydrate, uphold collagen, elastin and pass oxygen to the skin.

- Weather (Sun, cold and moisture);
  Already discussed sun damage to skin, however extreme heat and cold environment can also have similar effects. Damage to moisture can be seen in people who use harsh acne treatments over a period of time. Acne treatment dry out skin, it can cause damage similar to cold and sun, creating dry, tough, wrinkled skin as natural oils are depleted.

- Diet;
  Food that we eat can affect retaining a younger skin. Sugars, wheat, excessive dairy products, Processed foods and low intake of fresh vegetables and fruits creates inflammation in the body.

- Weight;
  Being too thin or too heavy can add to the aging process. People who suffer from eating disorders also tend to develop wrinkles dry skin and skeleton like features due to malnourished skin. Too much weight can case poor muscle tone, and sagging effect to the skin can show up due to weight fluctuation.

- Stress;
  High stress and Chronic pain in our lives can cause   our skin to reflect facial wrinkles.
  We frown, wince, and create a physical sign of our   stress and pain on our faces and body.

How can we Slow Down Aging?

Aging is inevitable. Good genes are one thing, but you can also help and age gracefully with healthy lifestyle choices;

Omega 3, 6 and 9
Finding foods rich in these Omega 3 are found in fish, nuts and flaxseed; Omega 6 is also known as Evening Primrose oil, Omega 9 found in animals fats and olive oil. They aid in boosting brain function, decrease inflammation, build and repair cell membranes, and aid with stress and hormonal management.

Water
Dehydration can cause fatigue, foggy thinking, headaches and constipation. The older we get the harder it becomes to absorb nutrients in the gut, and a hydrated gut is a healthier gut.

Food
Some foods are considered to slow down aging according to some researches. Foods loaded with antioxidants, healthy fats, water and essential nutrients combat dull complexions and fine lines.
Add the following into your diet: Watercress; Red bell pepper, Blue berries, papaya, Broccoli, Spinach, Avocado, Sweet potatoes, pomegranate seeds.
Cut back on Sugar.

Hormones
Most common hormone, the growth hormone and DHEA is responsible for aging, however progesterone, testosterone, estrogen and cortisol play a role in aging as well.
Our body's endocrine system secretes and controls Hormones that regulate many organ functions, metabolism, nutrient excretion and reproduction systems. These systems become less efficient, leading

to changes in our bodies, such as menopause. The hormone theory of aging states that these changes eventually cause the effect of aging. The Human Growth Hormone (HGH) has been found as a protentional fountain of youth, however research is indecisive on this.

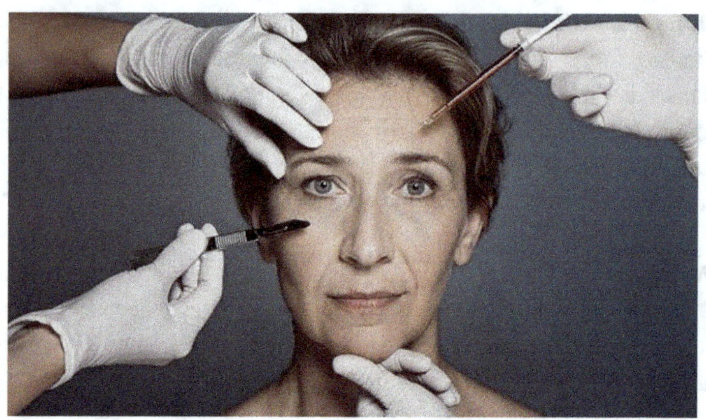

Chapter Eight - Product Knowledge

Understanding not all skin care products are created equal, as your skin is unique to you, so will your choice of products you use.

To understand products is to understand your skin type:

Normal Skin, is a term widely used to refer to well-balanced skin. A velvety soft and smooth texture with a radiant glow. Fine pores, good blood circulation with a fresh, rosy colour transparency with no blemishes and not prone to sensitivity

Oily Skin, describe a skin with heightened oil production. Oily skin tends to have blemishes. The skin has enlarged, clearly visible pores, glossy shine and thicker, pale skin and often blood vessels may be visible

Dry Skin, is typical less oil production and lack lipids that is needed to retain moisture and builds a protective shield against external influences. A rough and tight feel often more pronounced wrinkles and lines found

Combination Skin, varies in the T-zone and the cheeks. The T-Zone (forehead, down the nose and chin) appear oily and drier to normal skin found on the cheeks.

Other factors to consider when purchasing products is the age of your skin, colour and sensitivity.

Age; Our skin changes every 7 years on average. Oiler skin are found in teenage years can become drier post-puberty. Those with a normal skin type can find their skin getting drier. We lose volume and density; fine lines and wrinkles appear and changes in pigmentation. Skin also appear thinner as we age.

Skin Colour; ethnicity influences how our skin reacts to external forces such as the sun, pigmentation disorders irritation and inflammation. Basic skin colour is determined by the density of the epidermis and the distribution of melanin. Redness of skin is also measured of skin condition

 Sensitive skin is easily irritated by different factors which can be identified by redness, a rash, stinging, itching and burning. For some people high and low temperatures can also be a factor. It occurs when skins natural barrier function is compromised, causing water loss and allowing penetration of irritants

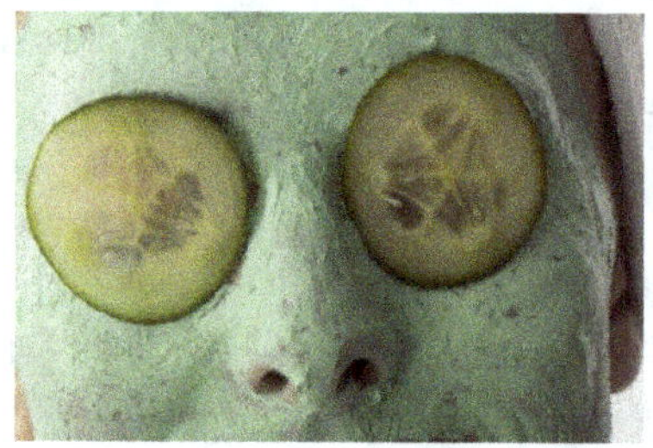

Estheticians use the Fitzpatrick Skin Chart to determine the reaction of skin to products they are wanting to use.

FITZPATRICK SKIN TYPE CHART

Please answer by circling the answer to each question

SCORE	0	1	2	3	4
Eye Colour	Light blue, green, grey	Blue grey or green	Blue	Dark Brown	Black Brown
Colour of non-exposed skin	Ivory White	Fair or pale	Beige with golden undertone	Olive or light brown	Dark brown or Black
Natural Hair Colour	Red to Strawberry Blond	Blonde	Dark blond, light Brown	Dark Brown	Black
Freckles on non-exposed skin	Many	Several	Few	Very few	None
Tanning depth	Not at all	Lightly	Moderately	Deeply	Naturally Dark
Face react to sun exposure	Very sensitive	Sensitive	Normal	Very resistant	Never had a problem

Total Score of all questions: ____________

Fitzpatrick Type	I	II	III	IV	V	VI
Total Score	0-6	7-12	13-18	20-24	>24	>24

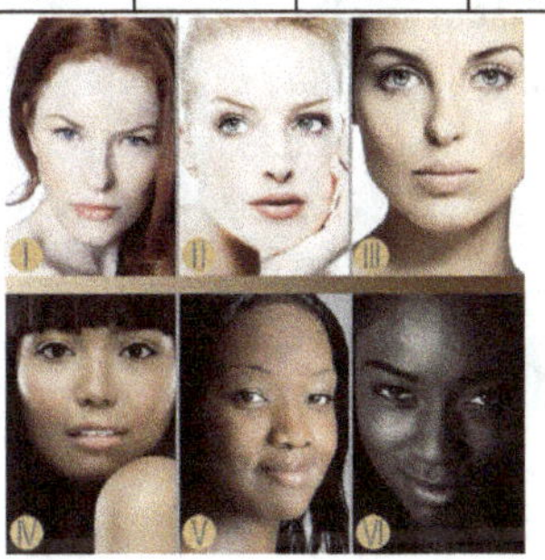

Chapter Nine - Skin Care Products

Buying the correct products for your unique skin can be a dauting task. You may also find this become expensive, especially when purchasing numerous incorrect products, ending up with cabinets filled with bottles, tubes and jars of products that caused your skin discomfort and break out.

Do not buy a product that claims to be for *All Skin Types*, you cannot use a product that is as effective for oily skin as it is for dry skin.

Cleansers: are found in soaps, gels, creams, milks and liquids, they are designed to remove dirt, oils, pollution and make up from our skin. Most cleansers compromise the pH level of the skin by adding ingredients such like, alcohol, acids and peroxides.
My suggestion is to use cleansers with natural ingredients like *TeeTree*® Oil.

Toners: If using a cleanser that does not affect the pH balance of the skin (eg; Clayton Shagal® cleansers) then toners will not be necessary, however, organic *Witch Hazel*® is a natural toner for the skin. Again, avoid Alcohol and Acids in the product.

Exfoliants: can come in Chemical (acids) or abrasive (oats) products. Do not use aggressive abrasive products like sugar, salt or apricot scrubs, they cause microscopic abrasions that can become infected or spread skin infections. Exfoliants should not be over used, less is more, once a week should be efficient, however, do discuss this with your esthetician as in some cases extra exfoliation can be beneficial.

Creams: are used to hydrate and protect your skin.

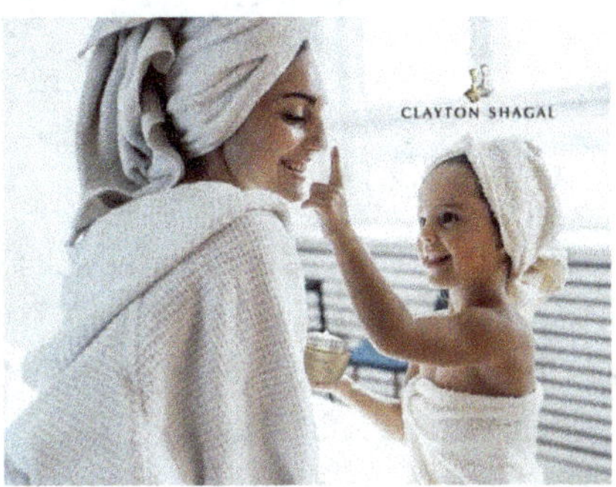

Collagen: Naturally found in the skin, however breaks down with age. To enhance these fibroblasts, some help in an Extract, Serum, Cream and or Gel. It can be injected into the skin and taken orally - harvested from fish and mammal proteins.

Used:

- to Stimulate formation of new collagen fibres in the dermis (upper layer of Skin);
- Accelerates healing of scars and burns;
- increase the skin ability to retain moisture;
- Delays formation of wrinkles;
- Works to improve the skin's foundation;
- Changes pigmentation of skin to be healthy and glowing.

Elastin: (synthetic and natural)
Similar to Collagen which is a protein found in our skin are also found in all mammals and fish however, can also be developed synthetically.

Used:

- improves moisture and elasticity of the skin;
- improves skin laxity firmness and tone;
- normalizes oily skin and skin carrying toxins;
- Reduces redness and inflammation.

Retinol: Is a vitamin A. A molecule, which is one of best vitamins for your skin. However, Retinol is known to thin down your skin with over-use, so be careful when you start showing signs of redness, flakiness, and irritation.

Used:

- It's a potent antioxidant and works to protect your skin from free radicals,
- Generates cell growth, and repairs damaged cells.
- Retinol is one of the only substances that is small enough to penetrate the outer layers of your skin and work its way down to the lower layers where collagen and elastin resides.

ACIDS

AHA: Alpha Hydroxy Acid. Not naturally found in the skin, it is however, a naturally occurring acid often referred to as fruit acids.

Used:

- used in cosmetic products as moisturizers emollients and exfoliants
- Also employed to treat such conditions as photo-damage, and hyper-pigmentation.

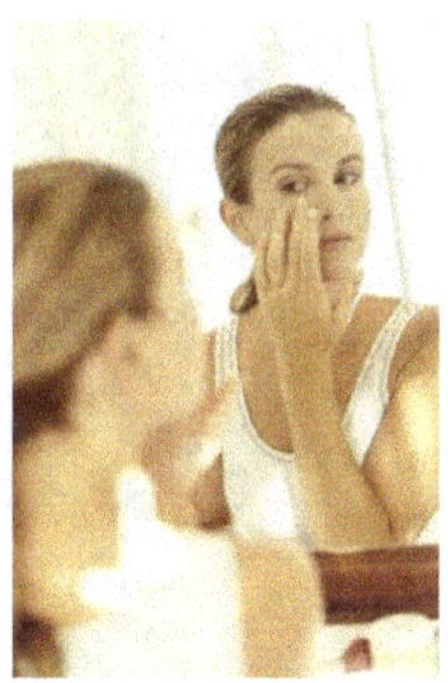

HA: Hyaluronic Acid is naturally produced in the skin to hold water in the tissue, like a sponge. These molecules can bind and attract up to 1000 times its own weight in water. It plays a key role in the scarring healing process, and in protecting against UV rays through its antioxidant action.

Glycolic acid, is not found naturally in the skin, it is typically derived from sugar cane, belongs to the alpha-hydroxy **acid** (AHA) family. Glycolic acid is known for its peeling effects resulting in exfoliating the skin from dead skin cells and oils.
along with malic and **lactic acids** — and is a common ingredient in many **skin** care products.

Salicylic acid is also not found naturally in the skin, it's a beta hydroxy acid which is found in fruits and vegetables.

Lactic Acid – is a weak acid found in Milk, it's specifically used to treat hyperpigmentation, age spots, and other factors that result in dull and uneven skin completions.

Chapter Ten - How Food influences the skin

What you put in your body, can result in good or bad effects on your skin.

The saying "you are what you eat", holds true to the effects it has. If your skin reacts then you know something you doing is not sitting well within your body.

I always refer clients to Naturopaths, nutritionists or their practitioners, that have bad skin reactions due to:

Allergies

Ailments

Acne

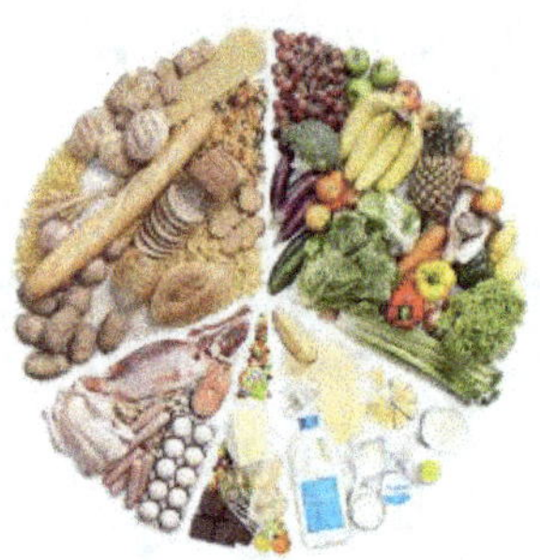

Major Health or skin   concerns are always referred to medical professionals.

I put a daily Food vs Skin quiz together to make it easy to eliminate the three main targets;
Wheat, Sugar and Milk. Fruits and starches (root vegetables) may also cause disruptions in our skin and digestive systems. If your guts are playing up with either constipation or diarrhea then it's a strong indication that your diet is wrong.

A very good documentary the Magic Pill®, is something you need to watch to understand some of the food crisis's we are facing.
Our food is now mass produced and to keep up with this production, farmers had to take steps to expedite harvests.

What do you think has happened to our food quality?
Take a tomato you have grown in your garden and compare the taste, structure and integrity with the tomato that has been supplied by your grocery store. It will surprise you.

Take the time and heal your body and skin with what you put in your mouth.

Record what you eat and where you broke out daily:

DAY 1	BREAKFAST	LUNCH	DINNER	BREAKOUT			
				FOREHEAD	CHEEKS	CHIN	AROUND EYE
WHEAT							
SUGAR							
MILK							
FRUIT							

DAY 2	BREAKFAST	LUNCH	DINNER	BREAKOUT			
				FOREHEAD	CHEEKS	CHIN	AROUND EYE
WHEAT							
SUGAR							
MILK							
FRUIT							

DAY 3	BREAKFAST	LUNCH	DINNER	BREAKOUT			
				FOREHEAD	CHEEKS	CHIN	AROUND EYE
WHEAT							
SUGAR							
MILK							
FRUIT							

Chapter Eleven - Hair Removal

To understand hair growth, will help you make the decision on how you would like to remove it. There are many factors to consider to keep you skin clear of hair.
It is also important to understand why the skin has hair, and removing it may cause other issues.

Hair Growth Stages:

Hair grows in four stages;
1. Anagen
2. Catagen
3. Telogen
4. Exogen

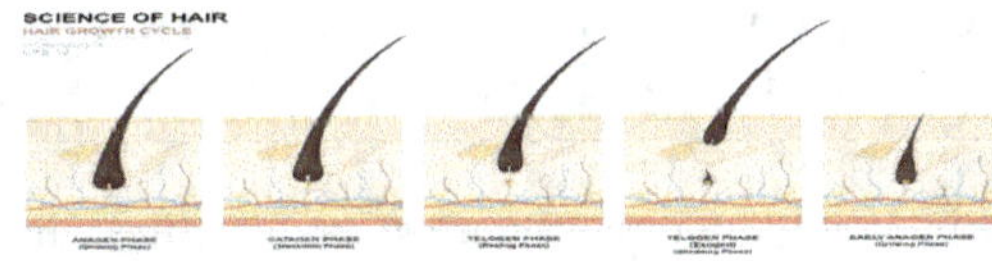

Anagen Stage:
Growing phase of the hair follicle, when the hair is in this phase the hair is the darkest, thickest and the healthiest. During this phase the hair grows about 1 cm every 28 days.

Catagen Stage:
The end of the Anagen stage, it signals the end of the active growth of the hair. In this stage the hair detaches itself from the blood supply (clubbing) and as it moves up and out of the skin, the hair follicle goes dormant. At this stage the hair does not easily fall out, except during exfoliating, combing, washing or hair removal processed (waxing). This process lasts for 2-3 weeks.

Telogen Stage:
This is also the resting stage of the hair follicle, at this point the follicle is dead, at this stage hair loss begins, you can lose about 50 to 100 strands of hair daily in this stage.

Exogen Stage:
Is also known as the Shedding Phase, as the dead hair follicle falls out a new hair is forming below and the Anagen phase starts again.

Purpose for Hair:

Hair is required to help protect the skin from Sun, environmental pollution and dirt entering the pores;
Hair by nature protects the skin, keeps the skin warm and/or cool depending how that hair is laying or the area it is found growing.
Cools the skin down, by trapping the sweat between the hairs on the surface of the skin;
When the skin is cold and goosebumps are form the hair stands on end to entrap body heat;

Waxing, Tweezing or Threading:

Home maintenance before and after waxing, tweezing or threading appointment.

Time:
For a better hair removal experience, it best to make you appointment late mornings or afternoons.
Mornings your body is still sensitive to evasive services due to skin dehydration.

In some cultures, and beliefs, it is said that hair removal just after a **full moon,** (Lower energy levels are recorded going towards the new moon), hair grows slower as the body energy slows down.

The body picks up cell regeneration and hair growth after the **new moon**, (Higher energy levels are recorded going towards the full moon).

In spring the hair starts shedding, and slows down in growth throughout the summer to keep the body cool;
In Autumn it starts thickening up and slows down in the 1st hair growth stage. This is the best time to Laser the hair as the hair is at its thickest and darkest.

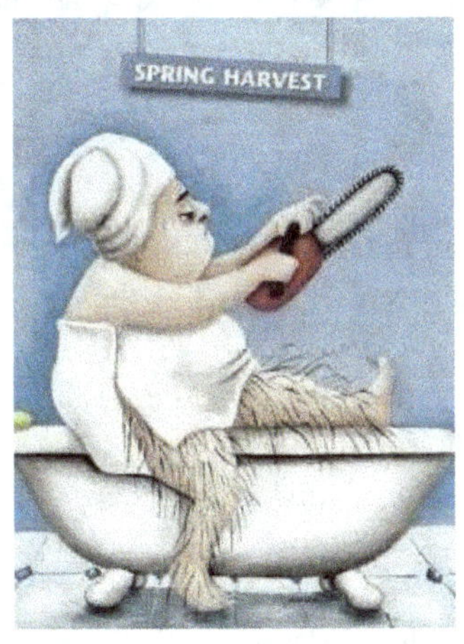

Hydration:
Make sure your body is hydrated (water);
Avoid, coffee, smoking (cannabis) or any other stimulus before a hair removal service.
When drinking water, it allows the skin cells to hydrate allowing the hair follicle to release from the roots easier.

Medication:
It is suggested to take an aspirin® before a service.
Check with your doctor /pharmacy about your prescribed medication
for hair removal services. E.g. Retinol, Accutane etc.

Hair Length:
Length of hair does make a difference in waxing, if it's too long the
pull of the wax will cause the skin to bruise, can also tangle and cause
hair not intending to be waxed pull and break off instead.
¾ of an inch is the ideal length and keeping the skin tight while
waxing, tweezing or threading does make a big difference in the hair
removal experience.

Results:
Keeping these tips in mind will lead to a better waxing experience,
however hair is still been ripped out of the skin and skin trauma is
inevitable.
Redness, light bruising, swelling, welting and in some cases bleeding
from the hair follicle is normal.
Ripping the skin off, deep bruising or blistering is not acceptable.

Ingrown hair.
I always suggest Which Hazel® be applied to the waxed area 12 hours
after waxing and then exfoliation with a coarse sponge or wash glove
within 24 hours also aids in the pores to stay open and allow the new
hair to grow.

LASER

Esthetic Laser Hair Removal, is not permanent as advertised on Social Media.
Laser hair removal is temporary and <u>reduces</u> the hair growth dramatically. You will find the hair follicle reduces in thickness, colour and finally in growth.
Once the hair stops growing, you will need to maintain this situation by doing Laser periodically.
There are various Laser machines out there and you will find various Laser procedures available, do your homework, ask questions.

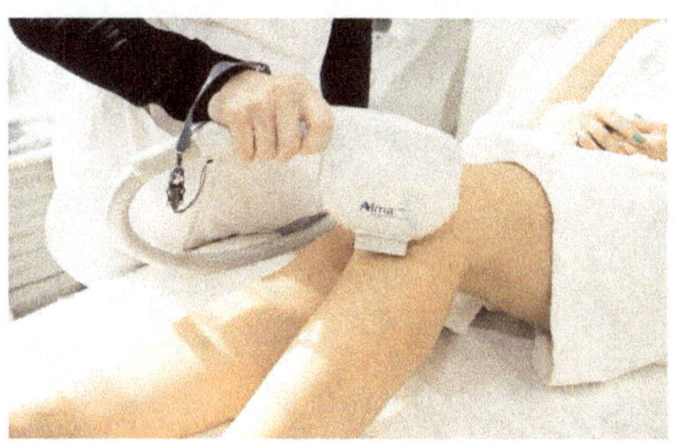

What you need to know:

- Laser does not work on blonde or light red hair, the best rule to remember when it comes to Laser, is if your hair is darker than your skin, then you qualify;

- You cannot do laser if you have any hormonal issues, medications or pregnant;

- Laser is for 18 years and older due to cell regeneration and Laser regulations;

- Hair may grow after child birth, Pre-menopause and post menopause, that is why it is important to do maintenance.

Notes:

Acknowledgments and references:

La Maison Clayton Shagal Inc.
Newsletters and Website
105-14056 Boul. Curé-Labelle
Mirabel, QC J7J 1L6

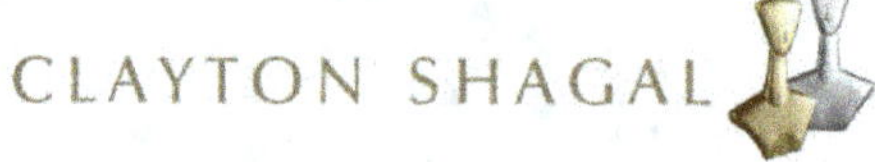

www.claytonshagal.ca